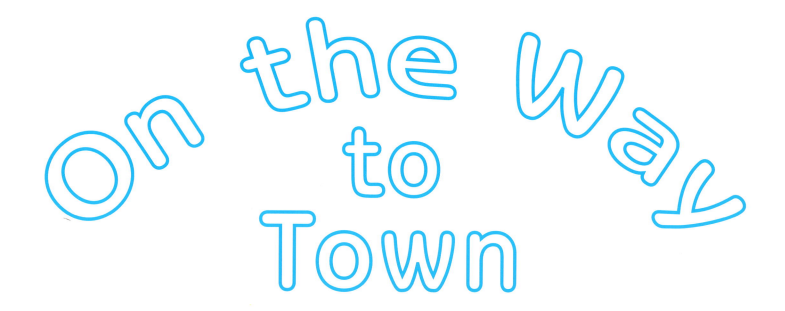

On the Way to Town

A road-user education book
for parents and young children

Written by Jean Roberts

Illustrated by Colin Hale

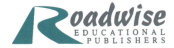

First published in Great Britain in 1995 by

Roadwise Educational Publishers
P O Box 4555
Halesowen West Midlands B63 4SY

Text Copyright © Jean Roberts 1995
Illustrations Copyright © Jean Roberts 1995
The Road Crossing Song © Jean Roberts 1995

British Cataloguing in Publication Data
A catalogue record for this book is available from the British Library

Printed in Great Britain by BPC Paulton Books Ltd Bristol

All rights reserved.
No part of this publication may be reprinted,
reproduced or transmitted in any form or by any means
(electronic, mechanical, photocopying, recording, video or otherwise)
without the prior written permission of the publisher.

ISBN 0 9524272 1 4

ON THE WAY TO TOWN

Introductions

    to the "On the Way" series of books   page 4

    to this book   page 5

a Story

    On the Way to Town   page 6

    look out for the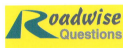

Questions

    relating to the use of Pelican crossings   page 27

and
a Song to sing   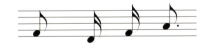

    chorus and one verse of The Road Crossing Song   page 30

An audio cassette and the "On the Way" Music Activity Book for Teachers are available.

The series of "On the Way" books are available from all good bookshops. In case of difficulty please contact the publishers direct.

Roadwise Educational Publishers PO Box 4555 Halesowen West Midlands B63 4SY

INTRODUCTION TO "ON THE WAY" BOOKS

Road accidents happen every day. On average over 30 children a day and 200 children a week aged 6 and under are injured on the roads in the United Kingdom; almost half are pedestrians.

How can accidents to children be prevented?

Children need to learn to make safe choices. If children are to learn how to cross a road safely for themselves they need to be involved in the decision making process from an early age: all too often children are passive participants in the road crossing process - decisions being made by adults with children just 'walked' across the road.

This series of four books illustrates different types of road crossings and how to use them. Safe crossing procedures are demonstrated in each story showing how children can be involved in decisions of where and when it is safe to cross the road. When out walking with a child and having to cross a road the same teaching guidelines as in the stories can be applied; and remember, when crossing a road always hold the hand of the child so that decisions can be checked before action is taken.

Each book includes questions within the story and questions with pictures at the end which will help to assess the young child's understanding. These may not necessarily be used the first time the book is read, but when thought appropriate.

There is also a song to accompany the series, a verse and chorus are included in each book. You will have the complete song when you have all four books. An audio cassette and the "On the Way" Music Activity Book for Teachers are available.

A small investment of buying and using all four books could save your child's life.

INTRODUCTION TO: ON THE WAY TO TOWN

When James and his mother went on a shopping trip to town they were amazed to see an elephant and a rather tall person......

This book has an interesting story designed to help adults and children know how to use Pelican crossings. However, it is not enough simply to think that a child has learnt how to cross a road using a Pelican crossing with just one shopping expedition. Children need plenty of practice. It may be that for some time the adult will say what to do - as in the first Pelican crossing example in this book. Next, a child may begin to respond - but not completely - rather like the response in the second Pelican crossing example - where the child recognises the green man sign and the 'bleep' sound and knows that he or she can cross - with care. Gradually the child will become more familiar with what to do when the light is on red (red man sign showing), green, or with the green man sign flashing on and off. The time taken for a child to learn what to do will vary from child to child. Children need to be questioned about their responses even when it seems that they understand, to make sure that they really are able to make safe decisions.

When using Pelican crossings the same questions as in this book can be used to help a child learn how to cross a road safely. To aid understanding there are **Roadwise Questions**

on some pages and at the end of the story there are more questions and pictures which can be used to explore the young child's understanding. These may not necessarily be used the first time the book is read, but when thought appropriate.

There is a song to accompany the series and the chorus and one verse is included in this book. Every book has a different verse and the song is complete when you have all four books.

Note: Some Pelican crossings do not have a bleep sound. This is normally when two Pelican crossings are used to cover a dual carriageway - when noise from one crossing could cause confusion at the other side of the road.

ON THE WAY TO TOWN

'Click' went the key in the door.

"Now you have your money for Sally's present so off we go," said James's mother.

James and his mother were going to town to buy a birthday present for James's sister and some clothes for James.

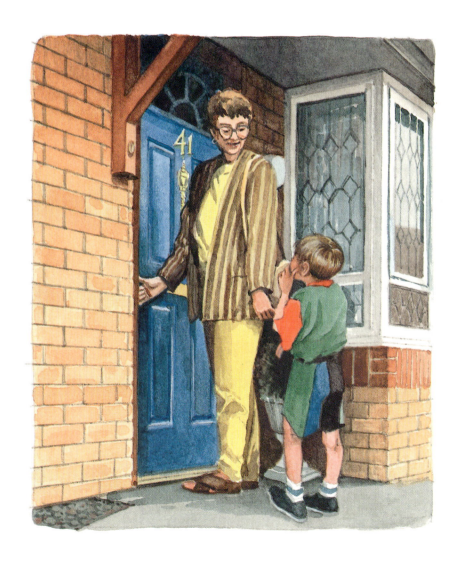

They walked up the road to the Pelican crossing.
"Look," said his mother "the light is red, we cannot cross the road now as cars and buses are moving. We will have to press the button. James, you press the button please."

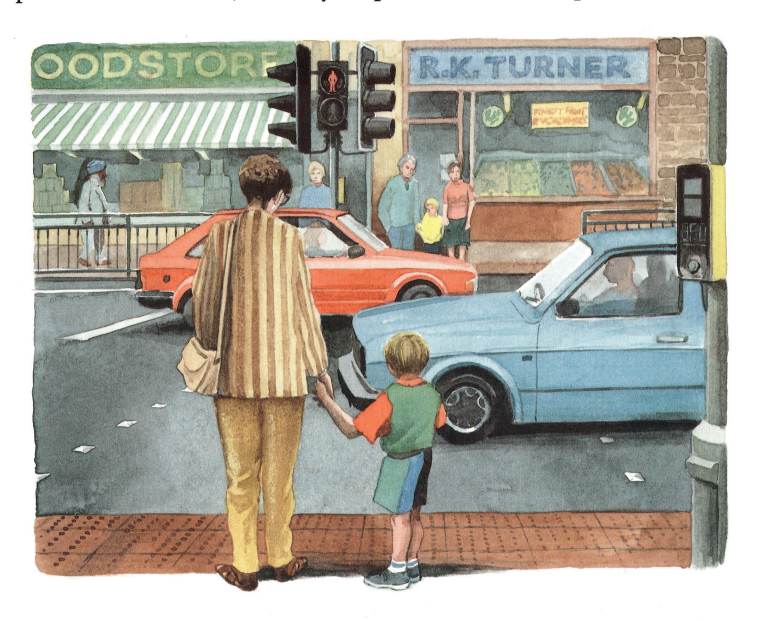

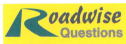 Can you see the red man sign?
Look out for it next time you cross the road using a Pelican crossing.
Where is the button for James to press?

James pressed the button and they waited.
"We must wait until the green man speaks to us with his 'bleepy' voice," said his mother.

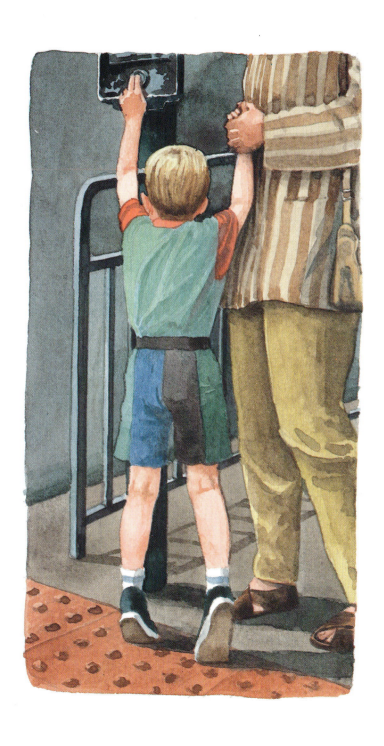

"Ah, now he's speaking to us with his 'bleep, bleep, bleep, bleepy' voice and saying that it is safe to cross the road. We will look all around and listen as we cross the road to make sure all the traffic has stopped and that nothing suddenly appears," said his mother.

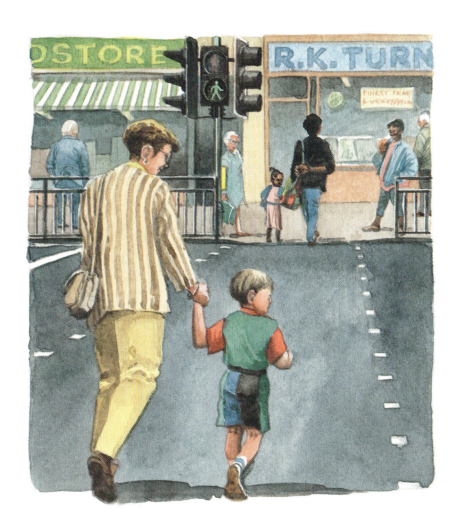

Roadwise Questions
Can you see the green man sign?
As we cross a road why do we need to look all around where traffic could be?

They walked to the bus stop and waited. It was not long before the bus arrived and they were on their way to town. James sat near the window and his mother asked him if he had any ideas about what he would like to buy his sister Sally for her birthday.

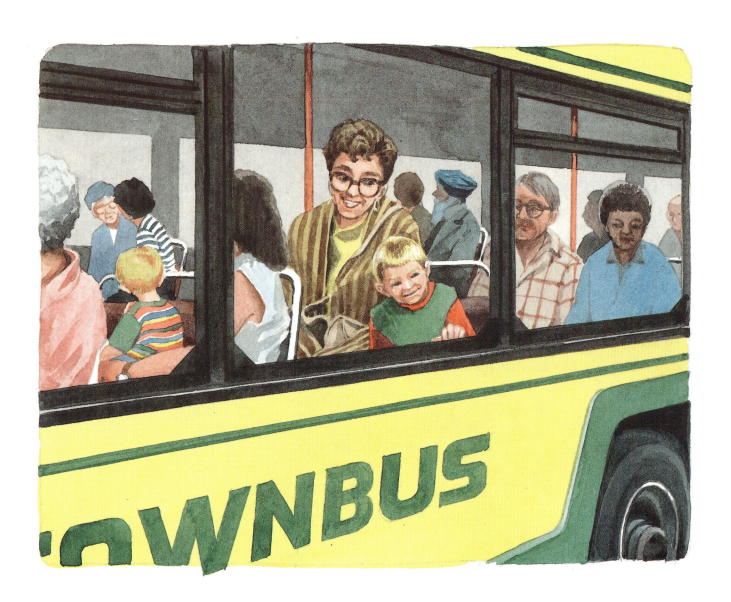

James was about to tell her when he suddenly shouted "I can see an elephant!"

James's mother was just looking for something in her handbag and without looking up said "James, it can't be: you're imagining it."

"But it is an elephant!" said James waving his arms around.

His mother looked up, astonished.

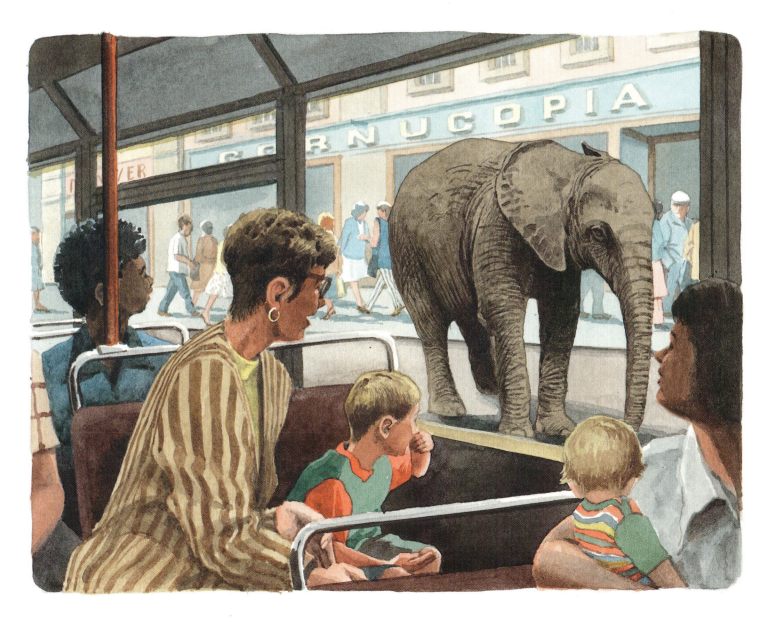

It was hard to believe, but there, in the town, was an elephant. "Well I never!" said his mother, "whatever next, an elephant in town! We shall have to walk up this way when we've done our shopping so maybe we will see the elephant again?"
James kept his nose pressed to the window while the bus went past the elephant.

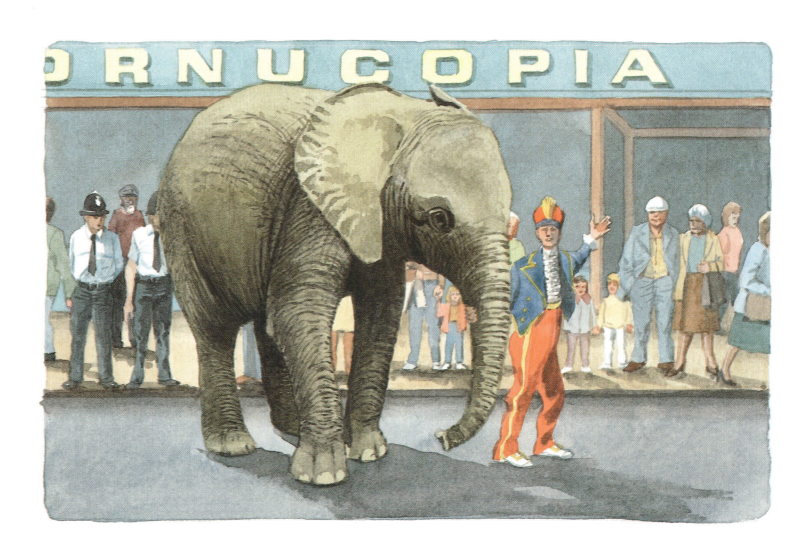

At the next stop they got off the bus and walked along the pavement. They had to cross the road so James and his mother walked towards the Pelican crossing. The red man was shining. "I'll press the button" said James. James pressed the button and they waited.

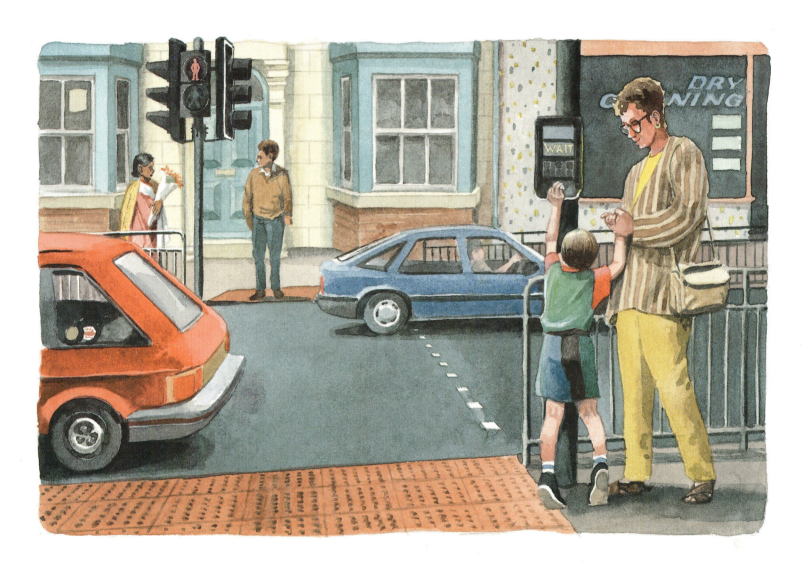

Roadwise Question: What will happen when James has pressed the button?

13

"How will we know when it is safe for us to cross the road?" asked James's mother.

James thought for a while and then the green man was shining at them and speaking in his 'bleepy' voice.

James quickly said, "Now we can cross the road."

"Yes" said his mother "and we must look and listen as we cross, just in case anything unexpected happens."

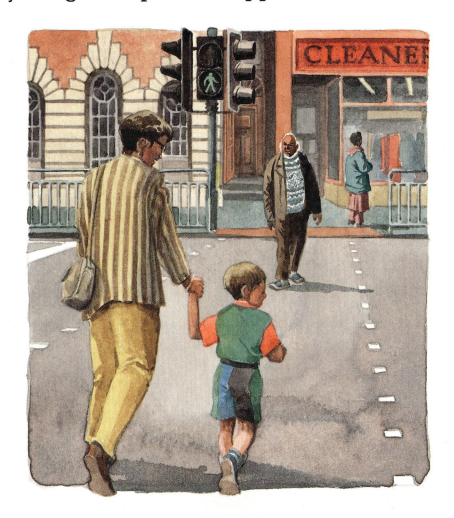

Roadwise Questions: What shows us that it is safe to cross the road?
Why do we look around and listen as we cross the road?

As they were crossing the road James noticed that the green man had stopped talking. He looked towards the light: it was going on and off quickly. His mother could feel James's hand tightening within hers. He looked around.

"He's stopped talking to us," said James "and he is going on and off."

"Yes," said his mother "but it is quite safe to carry on across the road as we are already on the crossing."

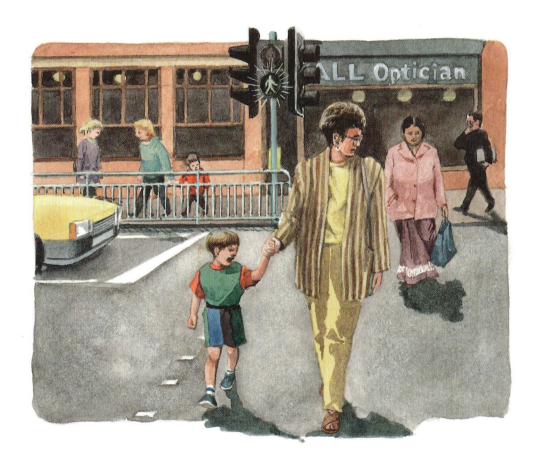

Roadwise Question When you are on the crossing, why is it safe to continue even if the green man sign begins to flash on and off?

They went into several shops and James could not make up his mind what to buy for Sally. Eventually they went into a lovely bookshop and James decided to buy Sally a book about animals as she was very fond of them.

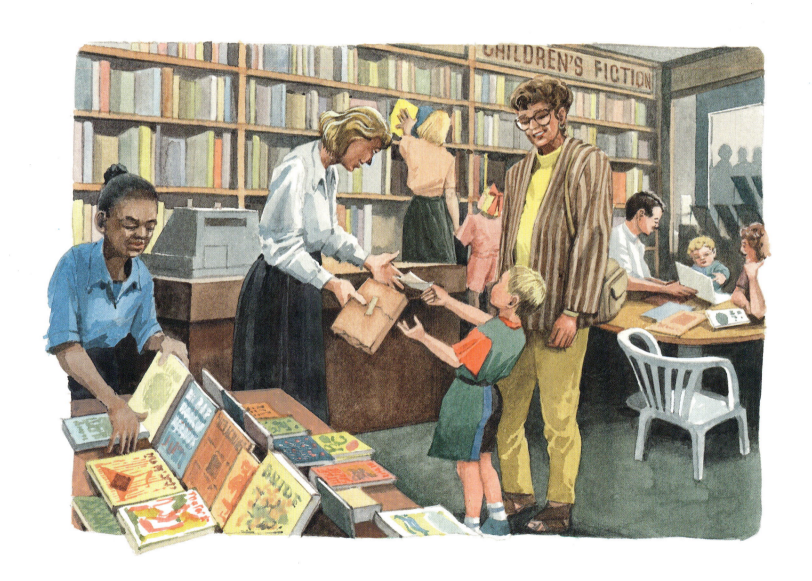

"Now I want to buy some new shorts and a tee shirt for you," said James's mother "so we will have to walk up the street and cross the road again. We shall be near to where we saw the elephant, I wonder if he will still be there?"

James spotted a Pelican crossing and said that they could cross the road there.

"Well done!" said his mother.

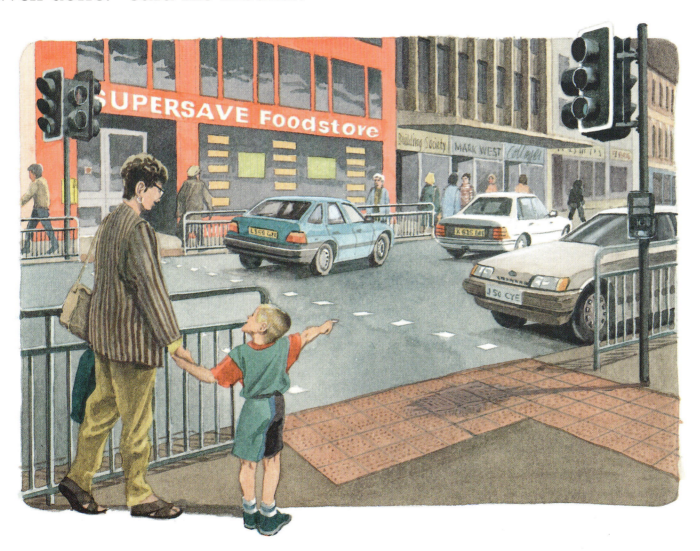

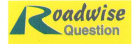 Can you see the Pelican crossing in the picture?

When they reached the Pelican crossing the green man was going on and off but he was not speaking to them.

"We can't cross now," said James "as he is not talking to us. The light is flashing on and off."

"That's right," said James's mother "what do we need to do?"

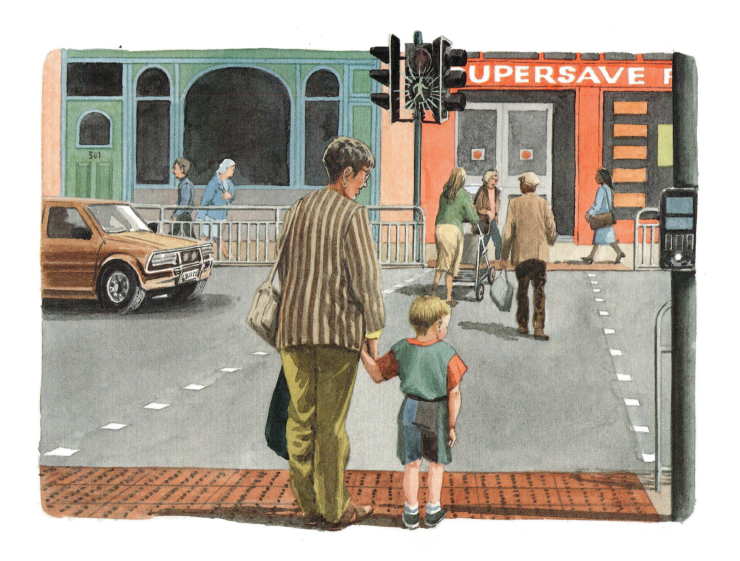

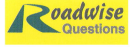 What should James do?
Why is it not safe to cross the road when the green man sign is going on and off?

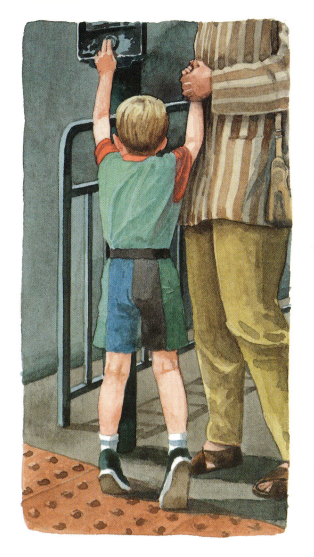

"Press the button," said James. "Well done James!" said his mother. James pressed the button and waited for the green man to speak to them. They waited.... and waited.

"What has gone wrong?" questioned James crossly. "Isn't he going to speak to us?"

"Look at all the cars rushing past," said his mother. "There needs to be time for the cars to be able to stop."

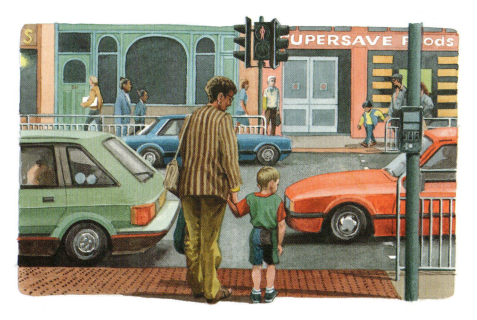

19

"Ah, there is his 'bleepy' voice at last. What must we do as we cross the road James?" said his mother.

"Look all around and listen to make sure that all the traffic has stopped," said James looking both ways and listening as they crossed the road.

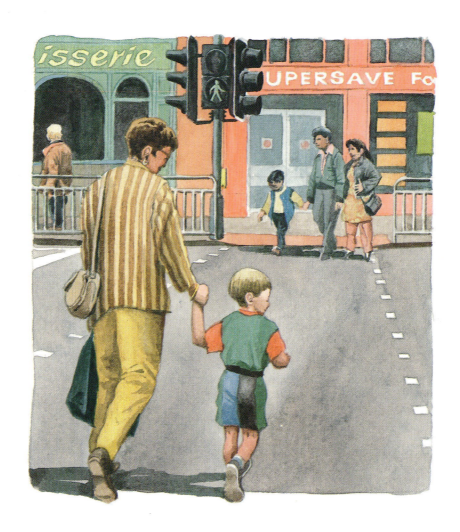

Roadwise Question: What must we always remember to do as we cross the road?

James and his mother soon found some bright shorts and a tee shirt for James. After they had paid for them they made their way to another door near to where they had seen the elephant from the bus.

Suddenly James shouted "Whatever is that?"
All he could see were some very large shoes and trousers that seemed to reach to the sky!

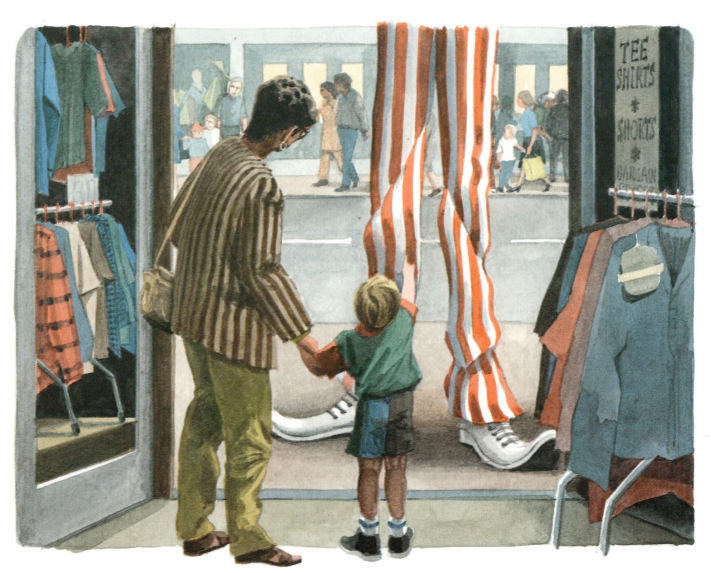

As they went out of the shop they were greeted by a very tall clown.

"Hello young chap!" said the clown as he raised his hat into the air.

"Hello," said James. "You are very tall."

"Yes," grinned the clown, "I can't get down to your height, but my friend here can."

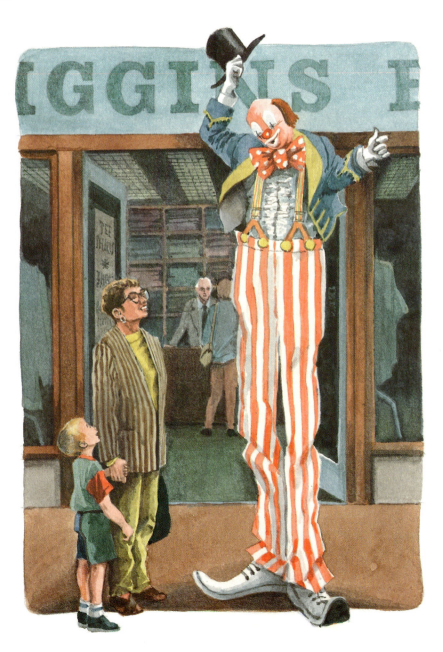

Immediately a very small clown came to say 'Hello' to James. "You can come and see us at the circus" said the little clown as he handed James's mother a leaflet.

"Thank you," said James and turning to his mother said "can we go to the circus please?"

"I should think we might," said his mother.

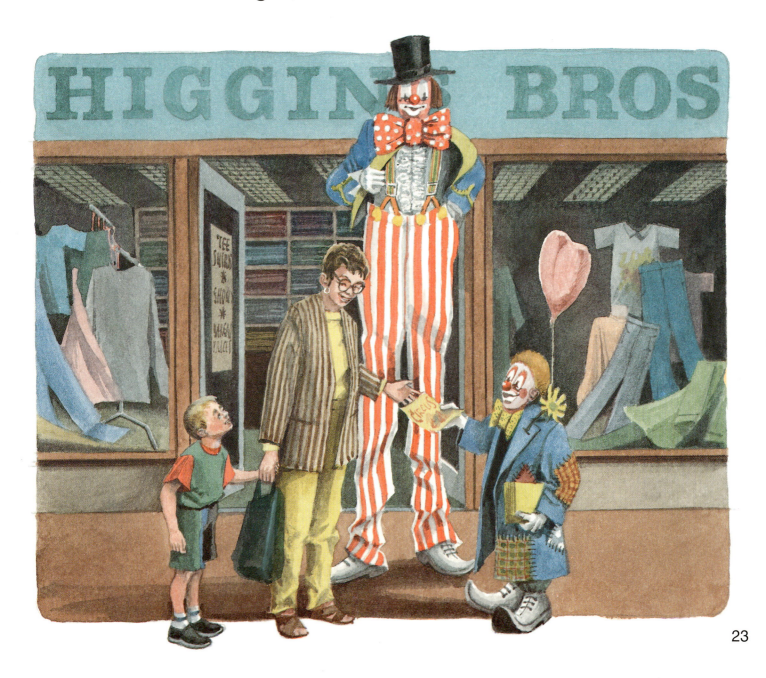

They watched the clowns for some time before they made their way to the bus stop and home. The bus stop was on the other side of the road so James looked for a Pelican crossing.

When they reached the Pelican crossing the red man was shining so James went to press the button.

"Well done," said his mother, "now what will happen?"

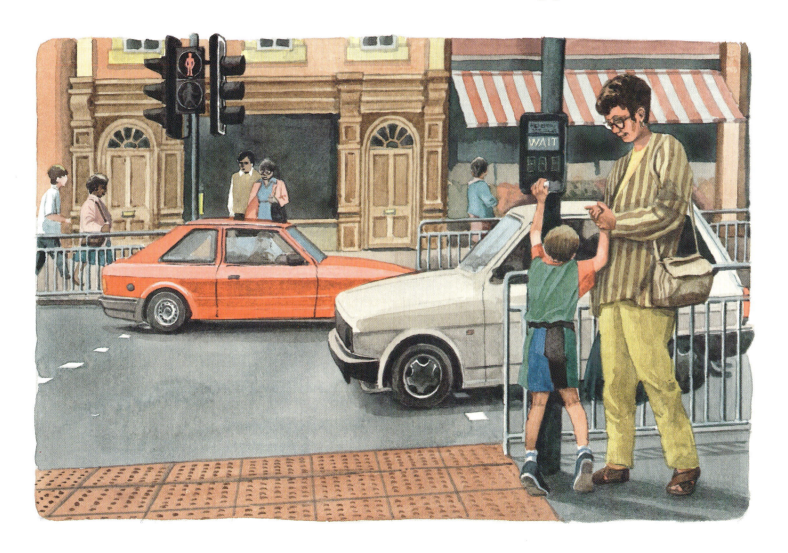

Roadwise Question What will happen next?

"The green man will shine and speak to us with his bleep, bleep, bleepy voice" said James. Just as he said that, the green man spoke to them and James and his mother crossed the road safely, looking and listening as they went.

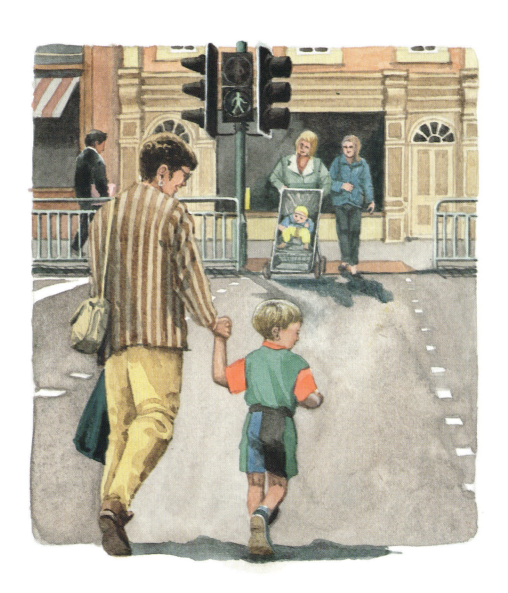

PICTURES RELATING TO USE OF PELICAN CROSSINGS

These questions can be used to stimulate discussion: to assess a child's responses the answers should be covered up.

In the story James was learning to cross a road using a Pelican crossing. When a red man sign is showing it is not safe to cross the road, the button should be pressed and then the green man sign will shine and there will probably be a bleeping sound. It is then safe to cross, but always look and listen when crossing a road.

Let's look at the story again.
One time when James and his mother were at a Pelican crossing the red man was shining.
What would you do if the red man were shining?

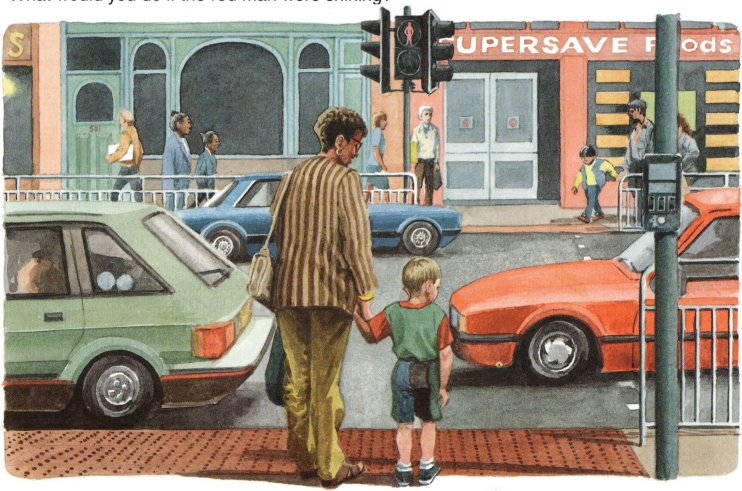

ANSWER   Press the button - just as James did in this picture.

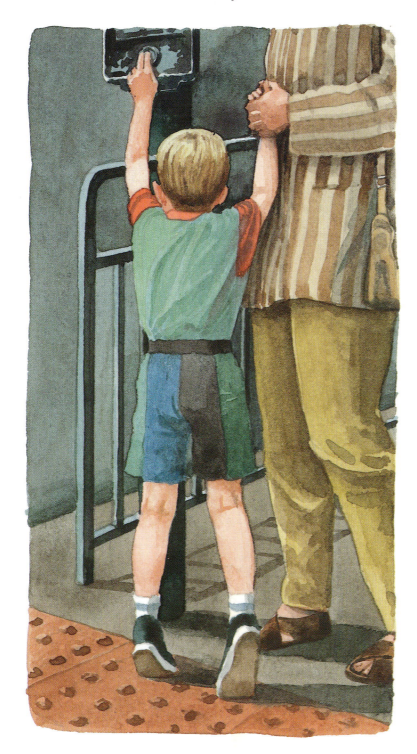

What will happen now?

ANSWER   The green man sign will shine and speak with his 'bleep, bleep, bleepy' voice.

27

What do we remember to do as we cross the road?

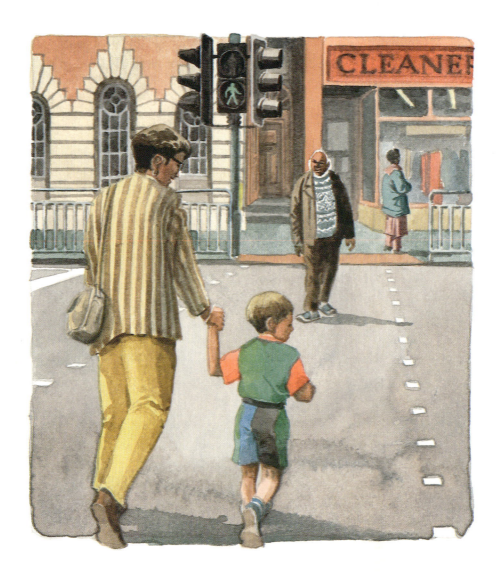

ANSWER   Always look and listen as you cross the road just as James and his mother did in this picture.

We should always look and listen when crossing a road in case something unexpected happens, maybe a car or bicycle will suddenly appear and you will need to keep looking and listening so that you can avoid having an accident.

One time when James and his mother were at a Pelican crossing the green man sign was flashing on and off and there weren't any 'bleep' sounds. If that happened to you, what would you do?

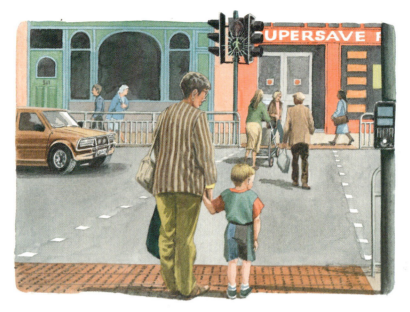

ANSWER   It is not safe to cross the road. We need to press the button and wait.

Look at this picture. What is there to help us cross the road.

Look and see:

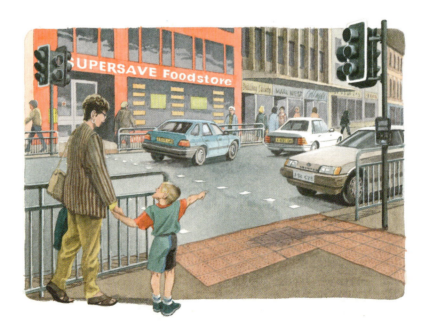

ANSWER   The Pelican crossing is a safe place to cross the road.

29

The Road Crossing Song

Chorus

© Words and Music by Jean Roberts
Arranged by Blodwen Roberts

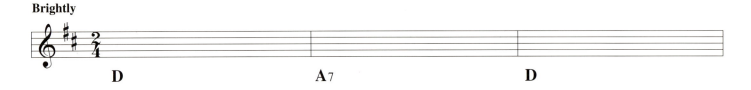
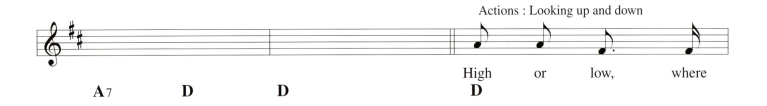
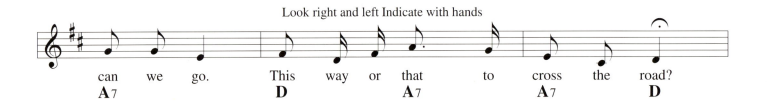
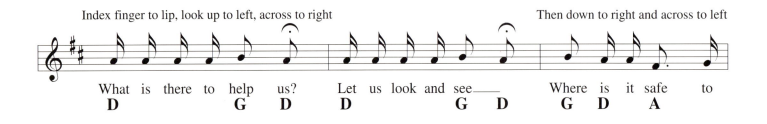
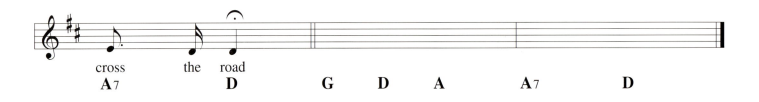

An audio cassette and the "On the Way" Music Activity Book for Teachers are available.

Verse

Spoken by reader of story, or teacher - " Is there a Pelican ? "
Response by child or pupils - " Yes ! "

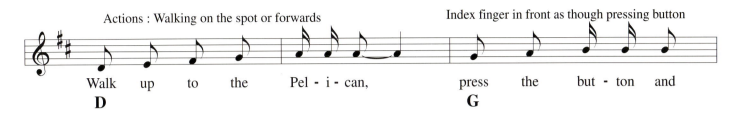

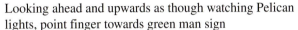

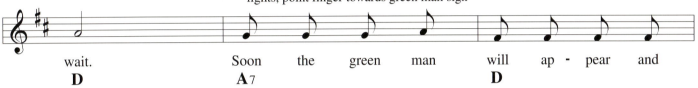

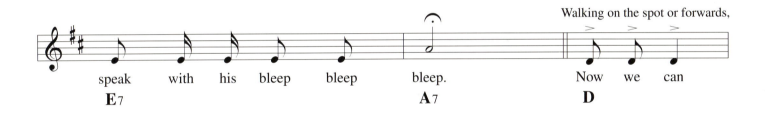

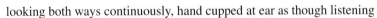

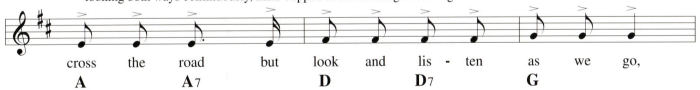

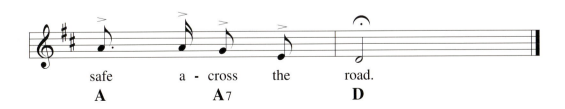

A different verse is included in each of the four books in the "On the Way" series.

31

Acknowledgements

Many people have given helpful advice by reading draft materials, spending time modelling for photographs, trialling materials in schools and helping in many other ways.

My special thanks to Margaret, Biddy, Winifred, Hilary, Eleanor, José and Arnie, Jennifer and Mitchell, David, Barbara, Don, Yvonne, Christine, the nursery unit at Benson Junior and Infant School and Tenterfields Primary School.

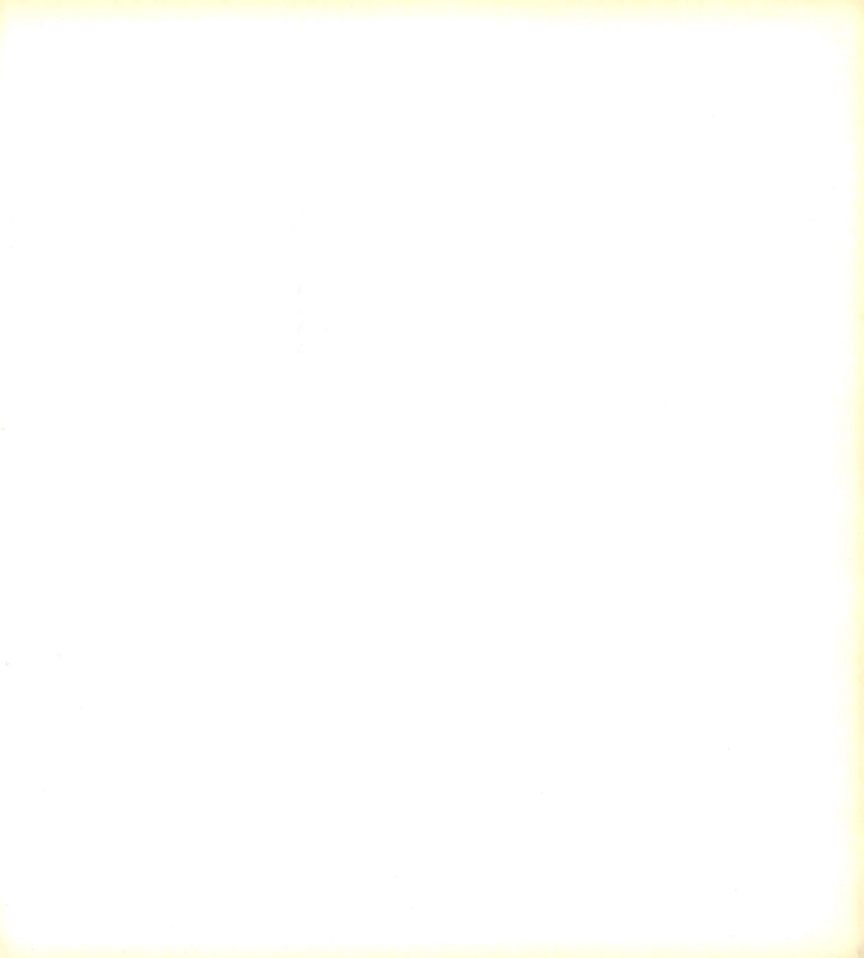